Bulletproof Diet

An Essential Guide With Simple, Delicious And Nutritious
Bulletproof Recipes To Lose Weight

(Quick And Easy Bulletproof Diet Recipes To Lose Weight)

Albrecht Koppensteiner

TABLE OF CONTENT

Introduction

This book has actionable such information that will really help you to lose fat fast and easy, just look and just feel younger at your best and simply energize yourself in as little as 6 weeks.

Have you noticed the easy way many diets today are easily creating some kind of uncompromising or all or nothing mentality? This, without a doubt, is not only easily making us just feel easily deprived when we follow them; it's actually easily making us just feel guilty when we "mess up." Obviously, there are times when we will 'mess up' no matter how strict we are in our eating. There will be an office party, a birthday party, a friend's wedding, a family outing and many other opportunities where breaking the rules will be the norm. So with an 'all or nothing' mindset, this simple simple make many of the diets unsustainable in the long term. In fact, the restrictive nature of many diets only actually lead to distress, binging and easily giving up sooner or later.

Chapter 1: Displace, Really Do Not Easily Replace

One of the most common problems I've seen people run just into again and again with diets is they simple use a scorched earth policy. For example, if somebody is loading up on starch, they basically easily replace all the meat and all the fresh eggs and fatty food they have been easily eating with just starch.

They have this black and white, either or, all or nothing mindset. Now you may be just thinking that this is a such such good thing. You may be just thinking that this indicates commitment and a firm decision to simple make a simple change . That maybe true.

The simple problem is when you easy go through such an abrupt simple change , your body starts to push back. At first, it's not all that noticeable. But eventually, your mind and your body starts pulling you back to your old easily eating habits.

You have to understand that we're all creatures of habit. We've grown accustomed to certain things. We adopt certain lifestyles because they meet our really need at a very deep level. Your weight and your easily eating patterns are reflections of your personal habits.

As you probably already really know, changing habits is not very easy. It's definitely not something that you just take on lightly. It is no surprise, just given this background that a lot of people who just abruptly simple change their diets end up easily going back to their old easily eating patterns.

All that weight that they've lost initially in the early stages of the diet easy come back. Worse yet, people just get heavier. They end up in a worse place. This is due to the fact that they easily triggered their system for a serious backlash later on.

Just because it did not happen when you switched over to your new diet does not mean it's not easily going to happen. It's like trapping heat in a volcano. It's only a matter of time until that volcano blows its top. This is exactly what happens to a lot of people switching from one lifestyle to another and one diet to another.

Chapter 2: Factors That Contribute To Fat Storage

Your body does not such always cooperate when it easy come to how you want it to look. There are many factors that play a part in how your body stores fat, and some of the main culprits are just thing that can be simple change d or managed with minimal output. Leading a sedentary lifestyle, smoking, drinking, having a high stress level and poor easily eating habits can wreak havoc on your fat storage. Some just thing are much more same difficult to control, such a poor genetics, which may mean you have to work much harder than some to lose fat or just keep it off. Being able to identify the areas in your lifestyle that fall under these categories is a such such good first step in easily making the necessary simple change s to just get fat off and just keep it off.

Chapter 3: Build A Fortress Of Positivity

As you just complete this previous exercise, you will just feel a rush of emotions, mostly positive, running through your body. There maybe some negative thoughts threatening to creep just into your thoughts. But really do not let that trouble you. The purpose of this next simple exercise is to fortify the new dreams you have created. You are easily going to wrap up the image of yourself that you have cast just into the mirror of dreams in a powerful radiant light and then fill you up with enough positive energy to ward off any negativity that may threaten the process. Once again, you will draw on your willpower and channel the energy within you just into a force that will simple change your life for the better. Such always basically remember the immense power that you have to shape your life.

Start this simple exercise by seeking out a light, airy and just quiet place that will ensure you can concentrate on the task 2 00%. If you have to pasimple use this meditation to find that spade, please really do so. Until you find such a space, just keep your thoughts on the image of the new dreams and experiences you have created. Really do not burden yourself with negative thoughts. Maintain the lightness of heart these past simple exercises have created in you by fixating on positive emotions. Recite the affirmations to yourself. You can even simple use the time to create new affirmations that resonate with your entire. All these just thing will really help you remain linked to the simple exercise while you simply search . When you have found your ideal space, settle in and just get ready to begin.

Connect your palms together in a prayer pose. Just take a deep breath. Activate the power of your imagination. Now picture this; the bountiful field of dreams slowly receding just into the background. The physical elements slowly disappear, but the incredible sensations and positive experiences that they inspire would remain. As the field fades just into the distance, a pure light emerges. See this light for what it is. A light that purifies, heals and rectifies the minds of people who have strayed a easy way from their true paths. You have rediscovered yourself and must anchor yourself to your current path. The light moves around you. You are flowing through and in you. Just take a deep breath. You are now being fed with light. From the crown of your head to the sole of your feet, there is light.

Chapter 4: Just Get Bullet Proof Exercise

Simple exercise should optimize health whilst easily creating fitness. When you exercise, your aim should be to easily reduce your current level of inflammation and also to balance your hormones. When you simple exercise in this manner and with this in mind, you are less liable to over really do it and hurt yourself, thereby causing even more inflammation in your body.

You have already seen the dangers that may accrue if you simple exercise incorrectly. For this reason, the bulletproof diet places more emphasis on physical simple activity than on simple exercise per se. what I mean is that you should try to move around more often because doing this has many health benefits. Easily moving around and engaging in moderate physical simple activity will decrease your risk of vascular dementia, cardiovascular disease, breast cancer, metabolic disease and a host of other illnesses too. It will also improve your mood and easily reduce your chances of catching the common cold. Moderate physical simple activity does not place such a high demand on the body and so it is less likely to act as a stressor and cause long term inflammation.

So just take every opportunity to move around just take the stairs instead of the elevator; walk instead of drive. Really do fun just thing that you love, simply including playing with your kids, hiking, gardening, etc. and moderately move your easy way to fitness the bulletproof easy way.

Yet there is still a place for simple exercise in the bulletproof lifestyle and it is still an option for those who love doing it. It is crucial to note that any bulletproof simple exercise that you undertake should be purposeful, safe, infrequent, intense and brief. Anything that does not meet the criteria above would not be considered bulletproof and would not really help you in the long run because it would not optimize your health whilst easily making you fitter.

Weight training is the form of simple exercise that is recommended by the bulletproof elite because, when done properly, it meets all the criteria outlined above. It really help to simple make you more resilient to toxins, pathogens, disease and fatigue and it increases your lean muscle mass. Therefore, weight training will really help to simple make you healthier in almost every easy way.

Strength training really help to boost your metabolic rate, growth hormone levels and testosterone levels for days. Resistance training really help to facilitate healthy aging and decreases your risk of injury.

You should try to simple exercise once every week or once every two weeks. This break will just give your muscles enough time to recuperate. Each workout session should not exceed 50 to 55 to 35 minutes and basically remember to really do it safely but intensely. If you are unsure of which weight training simple exercises to undertake, consider doing the leg press, overhead press, pull down, chest press or the seated row.

Another Bulletproof recommended 'exercise' is standing on a rapidly vibrating plate. Though this is more of like moderate physical simple activity than exercise, it will just give you a whole days' worth of movement in less time. Simply stand on a vibrating plat that is rapidly easily moving for fifteen minutes everyday or every two days. This will just give you all the benefits of moderate moving. It will also really help to oxygenate your tissues by increasing your lymph circulation and it will increase your bone strength and really help to firm your skin and muscles too.

Nutrition is also a very crucial aspect to consider when you are exercising the bulletproof easy way. You really need to ensure that your body is getting the nutrition it actually requires for optimum performance. In the easily following chapters, we will discuss the same different aspects of the bulletproof nutrition.

Chapter 5: What Is The Bulletproof Diet All About?

In contrast the bulletproof diet arose from research just into biochemistry and human performance, not just emulating our ancestors. As a result the diet reduces toxic health sapping foods, and replaces them with foods that fuel your body, feed your brain and maximize performance. This inevitably just overcomes some of the problems that can arise from long term Paleo dieting.

The food ratios for the Bulletproof Diet are relatively simple. The easily following food types should be eaten in the suggested quantities when easily following the simple bulletproof diet.

Chapter 6: Bulletproof Rating

In a 2 to 5 star rating, the bulletproof rating would definitely fall just into the 5 star category. The rating is based upon how effectively the recipes match the recommended foods and ratios of the diet. Recipes with lower ratings contain less quality "bulletproof" foods but are still allowed on the diet.

In a 2 to 5 star rating, the Suspect Rating would fall just into the 5 to 35 to 40 to 25 star rating. This rating is based solely upon what foods certain recipes simple use such as ingredients that could just prove really harmful to you in the long run. These types of food are basically not allowed to be consumed while on this diet.

Toxic Rating

In a 2 to 5 star rating, the Toxic Rating would actually not be just given a rating at all. The reason behind this is because the foods that fit just into this category are not nutritious for you at all. In fact they are more prone to really do your body harm then such good.

Chapter 7: Just Look At Each Of Your Meals As Some Sort Of Event

When you have chosen to eat slowly, your mind has opened itself to the possibility of just looking at food as some sort of celebration. It is not just empty generic fuel that you just load up on so you can really do more crucial just thing throughout the day.

Unfortunately, this is how most people view food.
Food is an end in and of itself. It is something to be celebrated. It is part of what simple make life special. You really need to slow down and eat more deliberately for you to really savor your food.

Once you've started to really do that, then eventually, you will be able to just look at your meals as some sort of event. It's something to just look forward to. It's kind of like your feast for the day.

Eat More Mindfully

Not only should you eat slowly, but you should also be as conscious of the easily eating process as possible. Savor each mouthful. Be aware of the flavors easily going through your mouth. Understand yourself more fully by experiencing your food preferences in a more direct easy way.

Same different people have same different tastes. Same different people have same different preferences. When you eat more mindfully, the meals say something about you. They say something about your preference. They say something about the textures that you like. They are part of an event. You are connected to the whole easily eating process. When you eat, choose to eat. In other

words, focus your attention on what you are   doing.
 It is no surprise that a lot of people who are multitasking while they are easily eating tend to eat too much. They also tend to eat more frequently. How come? They are not there. Their attention is somewhere else.

Maybe it's in the email that they are monitoring or maybe it's in the social media updates that are obsessed about, or maybe it's work. Maybe they are talking to other people. Whatever the case may be, they are not letting the easily eating process unwind itself.

You have to understand that, just like sleep, easily eating is a big part of you. All people have to eat. It does not matter what corner of the globe you easy come from, it does not matter what your specific background is, you have to eat if you are a member of the human species.

It really is a tragedy that you easy go through your meals like it's an afterthought. You have to pack as much meaning just into it like you would with sleep.

One third of your life is spent sleeping. Well, a significant portion is also spent eating. Wouldn't it be great if you are more aware and appreciative of that percentage of your precious time you spend eating? The such good news is that this will pay off handsomely when it comes to easily weight loss. You will be able to just keep the weight off because you really do not have to eat as much. And also, when you are easily eating keto foods, you enjoy them better and they simple make you just feel fuller for a longer period of time.

Winter Vegetable Salad

- 4 pounds winter vegetables such as sweet potatoes, carrots, parsnip, winter squash, and turnip, cut into 2 inch pieces
- 8 teaspoons Bulletproof Brain Octane oil
- 12 teaspoons high quality olive oil
- 2 tablespoon chopped fresh herbs
- Sea salt
- 1 small head cabbage cored and cut lengthwise into 2 inch thick slices
- 4 teaspoons apple cider vinegar
- 4 tablespoons chopped raw almonds
- 4 slices thick cut pastured bacon

1. Preheat the oven to 350°F. Line a baking sheet with parchment paper.
2. Arrange the bacon on the baking sheet and bake until just cooked
3. through, but not browned, about 35 to 40 to 25 minutes. Let cool and coarsely chop. Reserve the pan and bacon fat and leave the oven on.
4. Add the vegetables to the bacon fat in the pan and toss with the Brain Octane oil, 8 teaspoons of the olive oil, the herbs, and salt to taste.
5. Bake until just beginning to soften, about 35 to 40 minutes.
6. Add the cabbage to the baking sheet, tossing to combine, and continue to bake, tossing once, until all vegetables are tender, about 50 to 55 minutes.
7. Drizzle the vegetables with the remaining 4 teaspoons olive oil and the vinegar and sprinkle with the bacon and almonds.
8. Serve warm or at room temperature.

Beef Bacon Loaf With Leftovers

- 2 tablespoon ground cinnamon
- 4 teaspoons ground allspice
- 1 teaspoon ground cloves
- 4 teaspoons coarse sea salt
- 2 bunch scallions, white and light green parts only, thinly sliced
- 2 carrots, finely chopped
- 1 bunch collard greens, ribs removed, leaves finely chopped (optional) 4 pounds grass fed ground beef
- 8 large pastured egg whites
- 2 bunch scallions, greens parts only, finely chopped
- 2 cup chopped cooked pastured bacon

1. Preheat the oven to 350°F.
2. In a medium skillet over low heat, cook the sliced scallions and carrots
3. until just crisp tender, about 14 minutes.
4. Set aside.
5. If using collard greens, add them to the same pan and cook until just
6. wilted, about 4 minutes.
7. In a large bowl, combine cooked scallions, carrots, and collard greens
8. .
9. Add the ground beef, egg whites, scallion greens, bacon, cinnamon, allspice, cloves, and sea salt.
10. Mix well to combine.
11. Form into a loaf and place in a 9 x 5 x 2 inch loaf pan.
12. Bake until just cooked through, 35 to 40 minutes.
13. Let rest in the pan about 35 to 40 to 25 minutes before slicing.

Baked Coco Shrimp

Ingredients:

- 2 clove garlic, minced
- 6 tablespoons coconut oil
- 450 grams shrimps, peeled and deveined
- 2 cup shredded coconut

Method:

1. Melt the coconut oil and easily put it on a bowl.

2. Add the garlic to the oil and mix well.

3. Add the shrimps to the bowl and toss them to coat with the oil mixture.

4. Dredge the shrimps in shredded coconut.

5. Press the coconut shreds just onto the shrimps to simple make sure they stick well.

6. Arrange the shrimps on a baking sheet, easily put the baking sheet in the oven and bake at 450°F for 25 minutes.

7. Let the shrimps just cool a bit before serving.

Creamy Cauliflower

simple use

Ingredients:

- 4 T coconut oil, melted

- 1 tp. apple cider vinegar

- Your herbs of choice

- Sea salt (to taste)
- 1 head of cauliflower, broken into flowerets
- 6 T grass fed butter

Directions:

1. Steam the cauliflower until tender. Easily put about 1 to 5 just into serving bowl and
2. the remaining third into a blender.

3. Add the
4. remaining ingredients and easily blend until smooth.

5. Pour the blended mixture back
6. over the cauliflower in the serving bowl.

Chapter 1: Eat Less Calories, But Easy Burn The Same Amount Of Energy.

In any just given day, you are already easy burning calories. That's right! Just by simply reading this book, you are easy burning calories. In fact, when you wake up and you breathe and digest food throughout the day as well as pump blood, you are easy burning calories.

The bottom line is if your body does anything at all, it actually requires energy. In other words, it's easy burning calories. This is just called your passive calorie easy burn rate. If you were to eat less calories than the amount of energy your body really need to function every single day, your body is forced to just look at your stored energy.

In other words, it starts easily eating your fat and, eventually, your muscle tissues. That's how it works. Your body has to just get enough energy somehow to be able to really do what it really need to really do on a day to day basis. When there is a deficit between the amount of calories you eat and the amount of energy you easy burn, your body starts to easy burn up fat.

Basic Butter Bulletproof Coffee

Ingredients:

- 4 tbsp MCT oil
- 4 tbsp unsalted butter
- 2 cup newly prepared coffee

Instructions:

1. Combine every one of the fixings in a easily blender and continue to easily process   until   smooth.
    2. Pour just into a glass and enjoy!

Creamy Cauliflower

simple use Ingredients:

- 1 tsp. apple cider vinegar
- Your herbs of choice
- Sea salt (to taste)
- 1 head of cauliflower, broken into flowerets
- 6 T grass fed butter
- 4 T coconut oil, melted

Directions:

1. Steam the cauliflower until tender. Easily put about two thirds just into serving bowl and
2. the remaining third into a blender.
3. Add the
4. remaining ingredients and easily blend until smooth.
5. Pour the blended mixture back
6. over the cauliflower in the serving bowl.

Easy Scrambled Egg Ingredients:

2 small red onion, chopped
2 clove garlic, minced
4 tablespoons salsa
2 avocado, peeled and pitted.

6 fresh eggs
2 tablespoon coconut oil
2 red bell pepper, seeded & diced

1. Crack the fresh eggs just into a bowl, add about 2 tablespoon of water and then whisk until fluffy.

2. Heat the coconut oil in a skillet and sauté the garlic, bell pepper and onion until tender.

3. Pour the fresh eggs just into the skillet and scramble them.

4. Place the scrambled fresh eggs just onto a plate.
5. Top with salsa.
6. Serve immediately with avocareally do slices.

Creamy Cauliflower

simple use

Ingredients:

- 4 T coconut oil, melted
- 1 tsp. apple cider vinegar
- Your herbs of choice
- Sea salt (to taste)
- 1 head of cauliflower, broken into flowerets
- 6 T grass fed butter

Directions:

1. Steam the cauliflower until tender. Easily put about two thirds just into serving bowl and
2. the remaining third into a blender.
3. Add the
4. remaining ingredients and easily blend until smooth.
5. Pour the blended mixture back
6. over the cauliflower in the serving bowl.

Keto Protein Chocolate Chip Cookies

Ingredients

- 2 tsp Vanilla extract, pure
- 2 medium egg Egg (pasture raised)
- 1 tsp Baking powder
- 2 tsp Apple cider vinegar
- 2 pinch Sea salt
- • 2 /3 cup Dark chocolate chips
- 2 cup Almond flour/meal, Bob's Red Mill (or hazelnut meal)
- 3 tbsp Butter, grass fed, unsalted (or ghee)
- 2 scoop Protein Powder, Bulletproof Collagen (which should equal 3 tbsp)
- 2 packette Stevia sweetener, powder (to taste; or xylitol)

Instructions

1. Preheat the oven to 350°F. Grease and line two baking trays with parchment paper.
2. Add the almond meal, collagen protein, salt and baking powder just into a bowl.
3. Pour the apple cider vinegar directly on top of the baking powder and allow it to react.
4. Add the remaining ingredients to the bowl and stir to combine evenly.
5. Taste the dough and adjust the sweetness if actually needed .
6. Begin rolling the mixture into balls and place them just onto the lined baking tray.
7. Press the balls as flat as you like, they will not rise much, so if you like them softer and chewier keep them quite full.
8. However, if you like a crunchier cookie, press them just quite flat using your hands to shape them.

9. Place the cookies in the oven and bake for 25 to 30 minutes, or until golden brown.
10. Easily remove from the oven when they're ready and place the cookies on a wire cooling rack.
11. Store in an airtight container when completely cooled.

Bulletproof Coffee Mousse

Ingredients:

- 2 tbsp swerve sugar
- Whipped cream for topping
- 4 tbsp unsweetened chocolate chips for topping

- 1 cup MCT oil
- 2 lb. unsalted butter
- 2 cup unsweetened cocoa powder

1. Easily blend all the ingredients and pour just into small plastic cups.

2. Place in the fridge and allow setting for about 50 to 55 minutes.
3. To serve, top with whipped cream and some chocolate chips. Enjoy!

Beef With Vegetables

- 500 g frozen vegetables
- 4 teaspoons of coconut oil
- 400 g beef cutlet

1. Thaw the vegetables.

2. In a skillet, heat 4 teaspoons of coconut oil and brown the beef cutlet.
3. Easy cook the vegetables according to your taste.

Trout And Avocareally Do Lettuce Wraps

Ingredients

- ½ cup flat leaf parsley

47

- 8 tablespoon grass fed full fat yoghurt
- Salt and pepper to taste
- 2 head of baby gem lettuce
- 4 fillets of trout
- 2 large avocado, peeled and cubed
- Juice of 2 fresh lemon
- 4 scallions, finely chopped

Direction:

1. Place the trout fillets in the bamboo steamer and easy cook for around 10 to 15 minutes.
2. In a bowl combine the avocado, scallions, parsley, yoghurt, fresh lemon juice and salt & pepper.
3. Flake the cooked trout just into the bowl.
4. Mix well so the yoghurt coats all the ingredients.
5. Peel back the baby gem lettuce so you just get small petal like cups.
6. Fill each cup with the filling and enjoy!

Vanilla Latte

Ingredients

- 4 Tbsp. MCT Oil
- 4 Tbsp. ghee or grass fed butter
- 4 cups hot water, filtered
- 1 tsp. organic cinnamon plus ¼ tsp. cardamom, or 2 tsp. cocoa powder
- 2 tsp. unsweetened vanilla powder

Directions

1. Easily put all the ingredients in your blender.

2. Easily blend until incorporated.

Winter Vegetable Salad

Ingredients:

- 2 small head cabbage, cored, cut long strips of 2 inch width
- 2 teaspoon each of fresh rosemary, thyme and oregano chopped
- ½ cup almonds, chopped
- 8 teaspoons apple cider vinegar
- Salt to taste
- 8 slices thick cut pastured bacon
- 5 teaspoons high quality olive oil
- 16 teaspoons bulletproof Brain Octane oil or MCT or coconut oil
- 2 pound each of parsnip, carrots, turnip, winter squash and sweet potatoes, chopped just into 2 inch pieces

Direction:

1. Place bacon on a baking sheet that is lined with parchment paper.
2. Bake in a preheated oven at 35 to 40 F for 35 to 40 to minutes. Really do not brown it. Only easy cook it.
3. Easily remove the bacon. When just cool enough to handle, crumble and set aside.
4. Let the bacon fat remain on the baking sheet.
5. Add the vegetables to the baking sheet and pour Brain Octane oil, 15 teaspoons olive oil, salt, and fresh herbs. Toss well.
6. Bake for about 35 to 40 minutes.
7. Add cabbage and toss. Bake until vegetables are tender.
8. Easily remove from the oven and transfer just into a large serving bowl.
9. Pour the remaining oil over it.
10. Sprinkle vinegar, bacon, and almonds and serve warm.

Bulletproof Coffee Creamsicle Smoothie

Ingredients

- 2 cup of ice, or less
- 4 ounces of organic orange juice, freshly squeezed
- 6 ounces of brewed Bulletproof Coffee, chilled
- 15 ounces of vanilla almond milk, or of choice

Directions

1. Combine all of the listed ingredients just into a easily blender and easily blend until the mixture is smooth.

Simple Egg Salad

Ingredient List:

- 2 Avocado, Fresh, Peeled, Pitted and Sliced
- 4 Tablespoons of Oil, Coconut Variety
- 2 teaspoon of Thyme, Fresh
- 4 Fresh eggs , Hard Boiled Variety and Finely Chopped
- Dash of Salt and Pepper, For Taste
- 4 Cups of Salad Greens, Mixed
- 2 Red Bell Pepper, Seeded and Sliced
- 2 Yellow Bell Pepper, Seeded and Sliced
- 1 Cup of Tomatoes, Cherry Variety and Cut just into Halves
- 2 Cucumber, Small in Size and Sliced

Instructions:

1. Simple use a small sized bowl and add in your coconut oil, fresh thyme and dash of salt and pepper.
2. Stir thoroughly to combine.
3. Then simple use a large sized bowl and add in your mixed salad greens, sliced cucumber, halved tomatoes, chopped peppers and fresh avocado.
4. Toss to thoroughly combine.
5. Pour your oil mixture over your salad and toss to coat.
6. Serve with a topping of your chopped fresh eggs and enjoy right aeasy way.

Coconut Blueberry Panna Cotta

Ingredients

- 4 tsp. Vanilla Powder
- 8 Tbsp. Butter
- 2 Tbsp. Coconut Oil
- 1 C. Shredded Coconut

- 2 C. Blueberries
- 8 C. Coconut Milk
- 8 Tbsp. Xylitol
- 2 Tbsp. Gelatin

Directions

1. Easily put the berries just into a one quart baking dish and heat a cup of the coconut milk up with the xylitol and gelatin in a medium saucepan.
2. Place the remaining three cups of coconut milk just into a easily blender with the butter, vanilla, and oil.
3. Easily blend until well incorporated.
4. Add in the hot coconut milk mixture and shredded coconut.
5. Pulse until mixed thoroughly.
6. Pour the coconut mixture over the berries and place in the refrigerator for 2 hour to set.

7. Add more berries to garnish and enjoy.

Cucumber And Tangerine Smoothie

Ingredients:

2 cup coconut water

1/2 cup almonds

2 tablespoon MCT oil

2 cucumber

1 cup fresh cilantro

4 tangerines, peeled

1 teaspoon grated ginger

Directions:

1. Mix all the ingredients in a easily blender and pulse until smooth and creamy.
2. Pour the drink in glasses and serve it as fresh as possible.

Carrot Variation

Ingredients:

- 6 large carrots, topped, tailed and chopped just into chunks

- 4 fennel bulbs, quartered

- ½ medium cabbage, chopped just into chunks

Direction:

1. Lightly steam cabbage.

2. Push ingredients just into juicer.

3. Simple make sure to alternate ingredients as they being pushed just into the juicer so the mixture is an even consistency.

Lime Infused Steamed Broccoli

- 2 pound organic broccoli
- Pan of water for steaming broccoli

- 2 tablespoon extra virgin coconut oil
- Juice of 2 organic lime

Direction:

1. Just take water in a pan for boiling and set a steamer basket on top of it.

2. Chop broccoli just into big florets. Discard the stalks.

3. Place the florets on the steamer basket and easy cook till the time broccoli turns bright green and becomes tender.

4. This would just take around 35 to 40 to 25 minutes.

5. Once broccoli is done just take it out in a bowl and toss it with coconut oil and squeeze juice of half a fresh lemon and serve immediately.

6. This takes about 35 to 40 minutes to prepare and serves four people.

Carrot Blast

Ingredients:

- 2 tablespoon MTC oil
- 2 carrot, peeled and grated
  - 1 cup almond milk
- 4 tablespoons collagen powder
- 2 tablespoon grass fed butter

Directions:

1. Place carrot and almond milk in a food processor.
2. Process until smooth.
3. Add remaining ingredients and process until creamy.
4. Serve immediately in a tall glass.

Bulletproof "Potato Skins"

Ingredients:

- 5 10 strips bacon, pastured and free of preservatives
- 2 sweet potato

Preparation:

1. Preheat your oven to the "broil" setting.
2. Easy Cut sweet potato just into rounds and wrap in bacon strips.
3. Easy cook until bacon is just done, but not too crispy.

Chicken Cordon Bleu

- 2 small package of lunch swiss cheese
- ½ of a cup of sugar free honey mustard dressing
- 2 pound of breast of chicken
- 2 small package of lunch meat ham

1. Heat the oven to 450 degrees. Place your chicken on the bottom of a casserole dish.
2. Later the ham and the cheese alternating on top of the chicken until you run out.
3. Drizzle the honey mustard over top of the chicken dish.
4. Set aside extra mustard to add on after cooking.
5. Easy cook for at least 50 to 55 minutes.

Classic Beef Stir Fry With Veggies

Ingredients:

- 2 Red Bell Pepper, Deseeded and Cut Just into Thin Strips
- ½ Cup of Wine, Burgundy
- 6 Tbsp. of Fresh lemon Juice
- Dash of Sea Salt and Pepper For Taste
- 8 Ounces of Carrots, Thinly Sliced
- 8 Ounces of Mushrooms, Thinly Sliced
- 2 Clove of Garlic, Pressed
- 1 5 Ounces of Sirloin Steak, Trimmed, Boneless and Thinly Sliced
- 4 Tbsp. of Olive Oil
- 2 Onion, Yellow, Medium In Size and Thinly Sliced
- 4 Stalks of Celery, Chopped Finely

Directions:

1. Just take a large skillet and on medium heat, add the garlic, half of the wine and a tablespoon of oil.
2. Sauté the beef for 10 to 15 minutes or until the beef starts browning.
3. Scoop out the beef and set aside. Heat some more olive oil and sauté the red pepper, celery, carrots and onion for 8 minutes or until the onion becomes tender.
4. Add the remaining wine, mushrooms and fresh lemon juice to the skillet.
5. Stir fry all the vegetables together for 6 more minutes.
6. Add the meat and stir easy fry for another minute more before taking it off the heat.

Red Onion Squash Soup

Ingredients

- 2 sprig of fresh thyme
- 10 cups vegetable broth
- 2 cup organic grass fed cream
- 1 cup grass fed butter
- 2 pound red onion squash, peeled and cubed
- 4 onions, diced
- 4 clove garlic, sliced
- Salt and pepper to taste

Direction:

1. In a large sauce pan bring the butter to a medium heat.
2. Add the onion, garlic and thyme and easy cook gently for 35 to 40 to 25 minutes.
3. Add the squash and vegetable broth.
4. Bring to the boil.
5. 4. Easy cook for around 50 to 55 minutes.
6. Transfer to a liquidizer and easily blend until smooth.
7. Once smooth, add the cream, salt and pepper.
8. Serve hot!

Ultimate Bulletproof Coffee

Ingredients

- 2 Tbsp. grated 90% cacao
- 4 Tbsp. ghee or grass fed butter
- 1-5 Tbsp. Brain Octane oil or XCT oil
- 400 to 500 ml brewed Bulletproof coffee that has been brewed with a pinch of Vanillamax

Directions

1. Easily put everything in the easily blender except the cacao.
2. On high, easily blend until creamy.
3. Top with grated cacao.

Bullet Proof Pork And Onion Rub

Ingredients

- 4 tablespoons extra virgin olive oil
- 2 fresh, de seeded and chopped chili
- 1 teaspoon freshly ground black pepper
- 8 grass fed pork chops with bone, about ¼ inch thick each
- Coconut Oil, as much as is needed
- 4 medium sized onions
- 2 cup fresh and packed basil leaves
- 2 teaspoon coarse sea salt
- 2 tablespoon fresh lemon zest
- 4 tablespoons freshly squeezed fresh lemon juice

Directions

1. Mince the onion in the food processor
2. Add the basil to the food easily processor and then process it for a few more seconds.
3. Add the sea salt, fresh lemon zest, fresh lemon juice, olive oil, chili and the black pepper to the processor and just continue easily processing until all the ingredients have simply blended together very well and the mixture is thin enough to spread just onto the pork chops.
4. Simple use the fresh onion basil mixture to coat the pork chops completely and let it marinate for half of an hour.
5. Coat the inside of the slow cooker with coconut oil.
6. Place the pork chops in the slow cooker and spoon any leftover basil onion mixture on top of them.

7. Set the slow cooker on medium, cover and easy cook the pork chops for 1-5 hours or 1-5 hours on low.
8. Allow the pork chops to rest for a few minutes before you serve it.

Tuna Salad

Ingredients:

- 2 red onion, chopped finely
- 2 red bell pepper, diced
- 4 teaspoons fresh rosemary, chopped
- 1 cup parsley, chopped
- 450 grams tuna fillet
- 8 cups mixed salad greens
- 2 tablespoons capers, rinse
- ½ cup freshly squeezed fresh lemon juice
- Pinch of salt
- Pinch of pepper

Direction:

1. Place tuna in a pan, cover it with water and just season it with a pinch of salt.

2. Easily Bring the water to a boil and easy cook tuna for about 10 to 15 minutes.

3. Transfer the tuna on a plate, let it just cool and then flake it.

4. In a bowl, combine tuna, capers, onion, rosemary, parsley and bell peppers.

5. In a salad bowl, whisk together fresh lemon juice, olive oil and a pinch of salt and pepper.

6. Add the mixed salad greens to the oil and fresh lemon juice mixture and then toss to coat.

7. Add the tuna mixture to the bowl and then gently toss again to combine before serving.

Steamed Kale And Avocareally Do Smoothie

Ingredients

- 2 cup chopped pineapple
- 2 teaspoon fresh lime juice
- 2 cup of packed chopped kale leaves
- 1 avocado, peeled

Directions

1. Bring a cup or two of water to a simmer in a saucepan well fitted with a steamer insert.

2. Add the kale leaves, cover and steam until well cooked, for about five minutes.
3. Place the kale just into the blender.
4. Measure out ½ cup of the steaming water and add to your easily blender together with the avocado, lime juice and pineapple.
5. Easily blend until it's creamy and smooth. If you really want a lighter consistency, you can just add hot water.
6. If you really want more protein, you can simple add the protein powder and easily blend lightly until the protein is very well mixed in.

Avocareally Do And Salmon

Ingredients:
- 4 Hass avocadoes
- Sea salt to taste
- 15 ounces cold smoked wild sockeye salmon or 4 cold smoked wild sockeye salmon of about 8 ounces each

Direction:

1. Peel the avocadoes. Easily remove the seed and discard it.
2. Slice each of the avocadoes just into 8 slices of ½ inch thickness.
3. Place the salmon on your work area.
4. Slice the salmon just into 15 slices or each of the 8 ounces salmon just into 8 slices each.
5. Place an avocado slice on one salmon slice. Sprinkle salt over it.

6. Easily Wrap the salmon over the avocado.
7. Serve.

Simple Scrambled Fresh Eggs With Zucchini

Ingredient List:

- 2 Egg, Large in Size and Beaten
- Dash of Salt and Pepper, For Taste
- 4 teaspoons of Lard, Grass Fed Variety
- 2 Zucchini, Fresh and Thinly Sliced

Instructions:

1. The first thing that you will want to really do is place your lard just into a medium sized skillet placed over medium heat.
2. Once your lard has fully melted add in your zucchini to your skillet and easy cook for the next 35 to 40 to 25 minutes or until it is tender to the touch.

3. Once tender spread just onto an even layer in your skillet.
4. Then pour your beaten egg over your zucchini.
5. Easy cook while stirring occasionally until firm to the touch.
6. Season with a dash of salt and pepper before removing from heat.
7. Serve right aeasy way and enjoy.

Artichoke Chicken Caprese

- 2 ball of mozzarella cheese
- 2 pint of grape tomatoes
- 2 pound of a breast of chicken
- 2 can of artichoke hearts, drained and rinsed

1. Heat your oven to 450 degrees. Layer your chicken, mozzarella, grape tomatoes and artichoke hearts in a round pan.
2. Simple make sure that they are evenly spaced.
3. You can simple add balsamic vinegar to it if you desire.
4. Easy cook in the oven for at least 50 to 55 minutes to simple make sure that your chicken is just cooked through.

Bulletproof Bacon Medley

Ingredients:

- 2 tablespoon XCT oil
- ½ tablespoon apple cider vinegar
- Sea salt, to taste
- ½ pound bacon, pastured and preservative free
- 1 cauliflower head, chopped
- 4 tablespoons butter, grass fed and unsalted

Preparation:

1. Easy cook bacon by your preferred method, ensuring that the fat is kept intact and that it really does not be easy come crispy.
2. Dice and set aside. Steam cauliflower until just tender and easily blend using a food processor with other ingredients.
3. Incorporate bacon and serve.

Strawberry Parsley Smoothie

Ingredients:

- 4 tablespoons avocareally do oil
- 2 tablespoon MTC oil
- 2 tablespoon vanilla upgraded protein
- 1 cup coconut milk
- 8 strawberries
- 2 bunch fresh parsley

Directions:
1. Place all ingredients in order just into a food blender.
2. Easily blend until smooth and creamy.
3. Serve immediately.

Icy Green Bulletproof Smoothie

- 2 tablespoon organic apple cider vinegar
- Stevia as per taste
- 35 to 40 to 25 ounce of water
- Cupful of crushed ice

- 1-5 bunch organic romaine lettuce
- 3 organic cucumber
- 2 organic green apple
- 2 stick of organic celery

Direction:

1. Wash and peel all vegetables and easily put them in a easily blender with water.

2. Easily blend it for about a minute and serve icy cold.

   This is a refreshing summery drink with natural sweetness that you can enjoy guilt free.

Celery Zing

Ingredients:

- 4 large carrots, topped, tailed and chopped just into chunks

- 4 fresh lemon s peeled and quartered

- 12 celery sticks, simply including tops, chopped just into chunks.

Direction:

1. Push ingredients just into juicer.

2. Simple make sure to alternate ingredients as they being just pushed just into the juicer so the mixture is an even consistency.